Ruth Farrell
Ellie Walker
Sattar Alshryda

The Parents' Guide to Children's Orthopaedics

Slipped Upper Femoral Epiphysis

Ruth Farrell
Ellie Walker
Sattar Alshryda

The Parents' Guide to Children's Orthopaedics

Slipped Upper Femoral Epiphysis

Published by New Generation Publishing in 2017

Copyright © Ruth Farrell, Ellie Walker, Sattar Alshryda 2017

The author asserts the moral right under the Copyright, Designs and Patents Act 1988 to be identified as the author of this work.

All Rights reserved. No part of this publication may be reproduced, stored in a retrieval system or transmitted, in any form or by any means without the prior consent of the author, nor be otherwise circulated in any form of binding or cover other than that which it is published and without a similar condition being imposed on the subsequent purchaser.

www.newgeneration-publishing.com

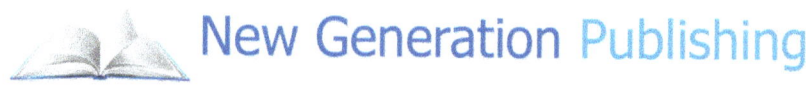

THE PARENTS' GUIDE TO CHILDREN'S ORTHOPAEDICS

Slipped Upper Femoral Epiphysis (SUFE)

Written by
Ellie Walker

(& Parents)

Series editors
Ruth Farrell

Sattar Alshryda

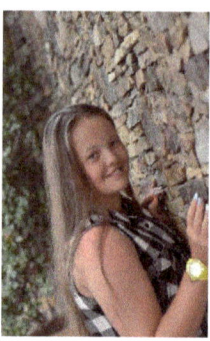

Ellie Mackenzie Walker
Ellie was born on the 5th February 2003. She resides with her parents Neil and Lisa, along with her 7-year-old sibling Isabelle Mae in Oldham, the UK.

Prior to her injury, Ellie was a very keen active rugby union player (since the age of 4), at the Huddersfield YMCA Rugby Union Club. She also accomplished her junior black belt status in Jujitsu at the age of 11.

Ellie is currently a Year 9 high school student at North Chadderton School, where she is starting to study for her GCSE's, in the hope of fulfilling her ultimate dream of becoming a veterinary surgeon when she is older.

Table 1 Table of contents

Introduction..	Page 1
So what is slipped upper femoral epiphysis?..	Page 1
Why does SUFE happen?..	Page 2
What are the symptoms of SUFE?..	Page 3
How is SUFE investigated?..	Page 6
How is SUFE classified?..	Page 9
How is SUFE treated?...	Page 9
How soon should my operation be performed?.....................................	Page 15
Should I have the other unaffected side pinned as well?.........................	Page 16
What about the recovery period?..	Page 18
What are the complications?..	Page 19
Should I ask for the screws to be removed in the future?........................	Page 35
Am I entitled for disability benefits?..	Page 37
Where can I get further information?...	Page 37
How can you help?...	Page 38
References	Page 39

Preface

Parents love their children and want them to be healthy and happy. They worry about them when something is not quite normal. Doctors are often consulted by worried parents about the way their children walk, the shape of their feet, their legs, pain, etc. They need reassurance that there is nothing wrong or if there is something wrong, for it to be investigated and dealt with timely and effectively. However, what is normal and abnormal is not always clear. This is particularly true for early childhood musculoskeletal developments and often doctors are not certain and advise a period of observation. This uncertainty triggers a vicious circle of anxiety which often results in exploring and further reading.

Although most paediatric units provide useful leaflets, the information provided is usually inadequate. The internet provides valuable resources for parents. We often direct parents to certain web sites to help them understand their children's problem. However, a significant number of parents find the amount and quality of information over the internet confusing and at times contradictory.

There is a lack of books/resources that provide parents with reliable information to help them understand their children's orthopaedic problems and get them actively involved in the proposed management in a way that positively influences the final outcome. Hence, we decided to start this book series project.

The Parent Guide for Children's Orthopaedics consists of a series of small booklets based on common paediatric orthopaedic problems. Each booklet is written by patients and parents to other patients and parents with the same condition. This is supported by the editorial team to ensure accuracy, comprehension and continuous update. The breadth and depth of knowledge will be set at what average parents need to know about that particular problem so that they can contribute affectively to their children's management. The frequently asked questions will be addressed in a lay person's language supported with evidence-based information that is explained in a simple way. Clinical photographs, charts and radiological pictures will be used appropriately to enhance understanding.

Some parents may find that some sections are technical and specialised, particularly when they read the book for the first time. They may find the information is overwhelming in certain topics such as the developmental dysplasia of the hips (DDH) and slipped upper femoral epiphysis (SUFE). Also some information may not be relevant for some parents and patients. It is our views that parents of today are more aware than previous generations and want to know more rather than less. They often read and know a lot about their children's conditions, sometime even more than the treating doctors! They often demand (and rightly so) the latest and the most successful treatments. We hope this book will empower patients and parents even more to work closely with the treating team to get the best outcomes for their children.

Ruth Farrell (editor)
Paediatric Specialist Nurse Practitioner
Royal Manchester Children's Hospital
Manchester
UK

Sattar Alshryda (editor)
Consultant Trauma and Orthopaedic Surgeon
Royal Manchester Children's Hospital
Manchester
UK

Acknowledgements

- We would like to thank all people who helped us through the various stages of writing this book. We are particularly grateful to Mrs Ania Milkowski, for her help in producing high quality art works for the book.

- We are grateful for the librarians of the Central Manchester University Hospitals for their support in obtaining published papers that have been used in this book.

- Authors and editors are really grateful for children and parents who have shared their experience with us namely Ms Lydia Gorman and Ms Charlie Greenwood.

Introduction

My name is Ellie Walker. I am 13 years old. I was diagnosed with a slipped upper femoral epiphysis 2 years ago, a condition that I had never heard of before. I was told that I would need surgery and that there were a few different types that I could have. Each has pros and cons. My parents (Lisa and Neil) and I were overwhelmed by the amount of information that we were given in order to choose the type of surgery that suited me best. We also read more about it over the internet, talked to various professionals, patients and parents. It was not a pleasant experience for anyone to go through but I am determined and positive that I would get over it and get my life back on track.

One thing that I really want to do is to share my and my parents experience with other people who are passing through the same situation. I hope this will help them understand the condition better, let them make the right decisions about their treatments and most importantly to be positive about it, as I was.

So what is slipped upper femoral epiphysis?

Slipped upper femoral epiphysis (SUFE or SCFE for short) is not a common condition, which is why most people have never heard of it. It affects the hip joint in growing children where the ball at the top (the epiphysis) of the femur (thighbone) slips away from the rest of the bone. Imagine the top of your femur being like a baseball that has been cut in half, with a piece of soft material/jelly (the growth plate) in the middle that enables children to grow. The top half of the baseball has slipped off the bottom half (Figure 1). This usually develops gradually over time. However, it could happen very quickly - a fall or a trip may speed it up. If you are unfortunate, the blood vessels that feed the ball of the joint may get cut off when it slips away from the rest of femur. This will cause the ball of the joint to die and disappear. Doctors call this "avascular necrosis" of the femoral head, or AVN for short (more on this later).

Figure 1 Slipped upper femoral epiphysis

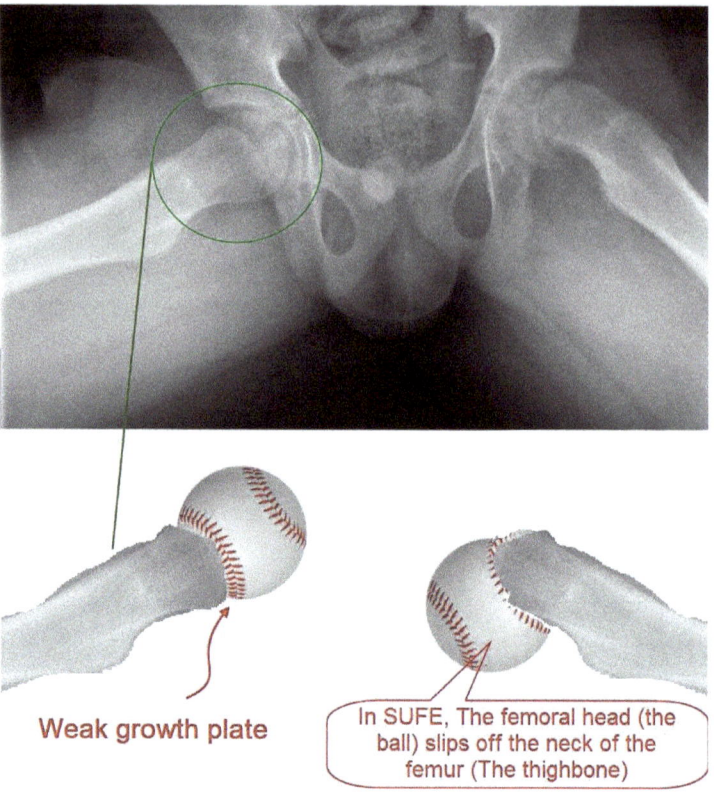

SUFE is called acute if it occurs over a 3 week period and chronic if it occurs over a longer period. Some chronic SUFE become acute when further slipping happens over a very short period of time. This type of SUFE is often called acute-on-chronic slip.

Why does SUFE happen?

Nobody knows exactly why SUFE happens. However, it is assumed that either the growth plate (the soft material between the two halves of the baseball!) is weaker than normal or there is an excessive force that breaks the growth plate. This is probably the reason why it is more common in overweight children.

Several conditions are known to cause a weak growth plate such as kidney failure and growth and thyroid hormone disorders. I did not have any of these disorders and my doctor said that this is the case in most children who are diagnosed with SUFE. This type of SUFE, when no cause has been identified, is often called idiopathic. There is a test called the "age-weight test" that can predict whether the slip is idiopathic or not (i.e. there is an underlying disorder that has caused the slip). As the name implies, the test is based on patient's age and weight. When the test is negative, the chance of having an idiopathic SUFE is around 90%. However, when the test is positive, there is 50% chance that the slip is due to an underlying condition [1].

What are the symptoms of SUFE?

Symptoms of SUFE vary from patient to patient. In stable SUFE, symptoms are usually mild and intermittent pain in the groin, thigh and/or knee. This may last for several weeks or months. The pain is usually made worse by doing sports and physical activities. Friends and family may notice that you have started limping. You may also notice that the affected leg is pointing outward more than your other leg (Figure 2).

Sometimes the symptoms are so mild that the affected person may never seek medical advice. My dad was told that he probably had SUFE when he was a child but never sought medical advice. Now, he complains of bad hip pain and he was told that he would need a hip replacement. Doctors explained that his hips on X-ray look like a pistol grip and this is how hips with healed SUFE look on plain X-rays (Figure 3).

Figure 2 Clinical photograph of a child with left SUFE

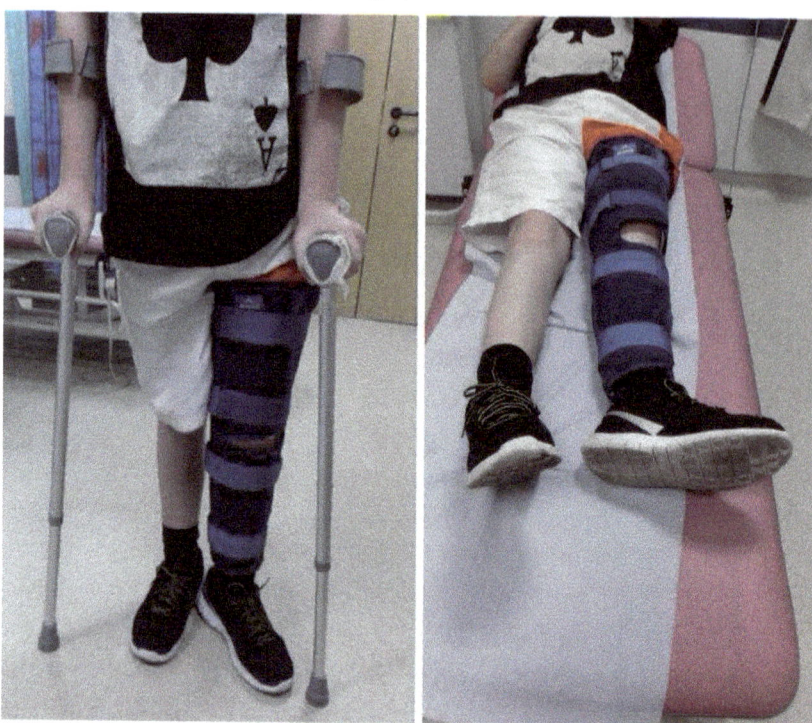

It is not unusual that a child with SUFE complains of knee pain mainly. This child had been investigated and treated for knee pain despite the cause of his knee pain being a slipped upper femoral epiphysis

Figure 3 Healed mild slipped upper femoral epiphysis

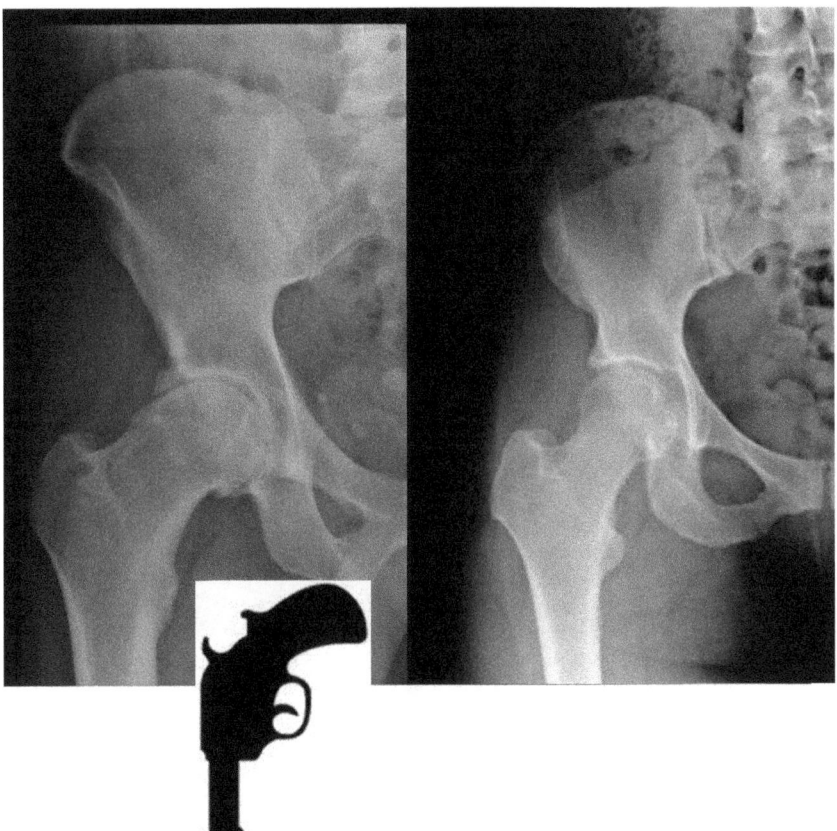

Pistol grip appearance of healed mild SUFE (left image) in comparison to the normal appearance of the hip (right image).

If you have an unstable SUFE, symptoms are usually more pronounced. Pain is usually sudden and may follow a fall or a trip. You may not be able to walk, stand or even lift your leg. You may notice that the leg is short and turned outward (Figure 4).

The earlier you seek advice the better. My doctor told me that it is sad that most patients and parents dismiss the initial symptoms and do not attend until the slip becomes moderate to severe.

Figure 4 a patient with unstable SUFE

The left leg is turning outward. This child was brought to hospital on a stretcher and he was not able even to stand.

How is SUFE investigated?

My doctor ordered an X-ray of the hips from different angles to confirm that I had a SUFE and he measured several angles on the X-ray to determine the severity of the slip. There are 3 grades of severity based on how far the ball tilted away from the rest of the thigh bone. These are mild, moderate and severe (Figure 5).

Figure 5 Grades of slip severity

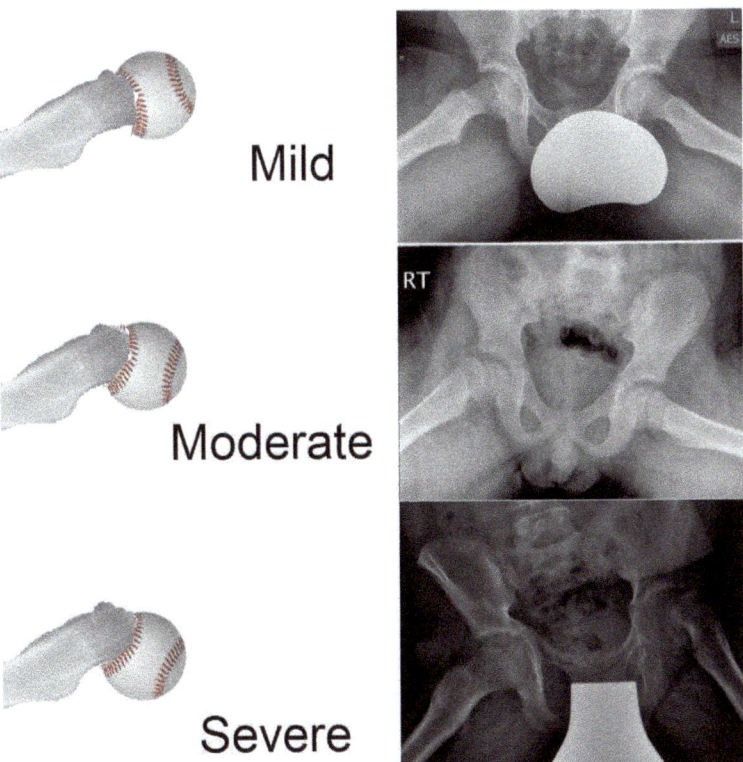

The plain X-ray is usually sufficient to confirm the diagnosis and plan the treatment. However, there are occasions when further tests are required:

1. When the slip is very mild or early (this is called a pre-slip). With X-ray alone, it is not possible to be certain that there is a slip. Magnetic resonance imaging (MRI) can confirm the presence of a slip and also rule out other causes of pain (Figure 6).

2. If the slip is severe and your doctor is considering an operation to correct it, your doctor may order a CT (computed tomography) scan and/or MRI scan. Both these radiological tests give more information about the slip and whether you have developed an AVN. The CT scan provides surgeons with a three dimensional view of your hip. This helps in assessing the severity of deformity better and enables your doctor to choose the right procedure and metal implant to stabilise the slip.

3. Blood tests are ordered when an underlying disorder is suspected such as kidney disease or hormonal imbalance (see above). They may also be requested by the anaesthetist in preparation for surgery.

Figure 6 MRI scan confirming SUFE when the X-ray could not

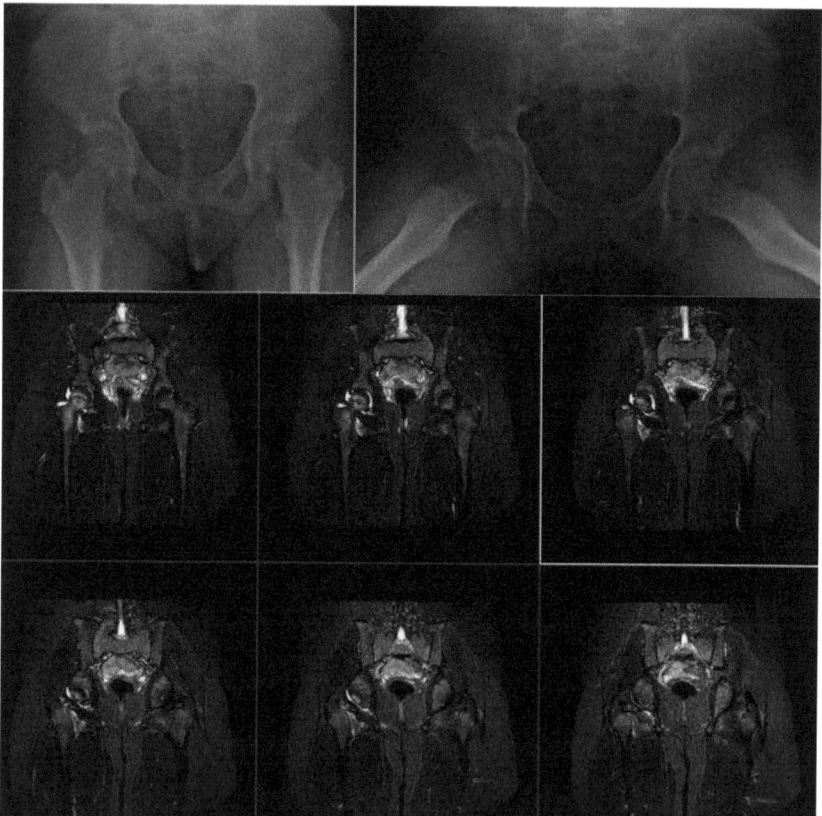

The plain X-ray did not show a slip; however, the MRI scan showed a high signal at the growth plate (the growth plate looks whiter than the other side) indicating there is breaking of the growth plate.

How is SUFE classified?

SUFE can be classified in different ways. I mentioned earlier that SUFE can be mild, moderate or severe based on the severity of the slip. It can also be acute, chronic or acute on chronic, based on the duration of symptoms.

However, classifying the slip into stable and unstable is the most useful classification as it is closely related to the future outcome [2, 3]. A slip is considered to be **stable** when sufferers are able to walk and bear their weight, even if it means they need crutches to do so, whereas the slip is considered to be **unstable** when they are unable to walk even with crutches. About 50% of children with unstable slips develop AVN of the femoral head [4]. The risk of developing AVN in children with a stable slip is around 2%. Femoral head AVN is closely related to the future outcome of SUFE. Most studies have used AVN as indicator for poor outcome.

The femoral head AVN is not unique to unstable SUFE. It is also seen in several other conditions such as femoral neck fractures, sickle cell disease and following treatment of dislocated hips. The reason behind this is that the arterial supply to the femoral head is well fixed to the femoral neck and is easily damaged with any femoral neck fracture displacement or sudden slip contrary to gradual displacement in stable slip. Furthermore, nutrient vessels going to the femoral head terminate as small arterioles that are easily occluded with small thrombi (blood clots). This happens in sickle cell disease and steroid treatment.

How is SUFE treated?

Once SUFE is confirmed, surgery is required to prevent progression of the slip and allow return to walking. For the same reason, you will not be allowed to bear weight and will probably be admitted to the hospital on the same day. The type of operation that your doctor recommends will depend upon the severity of the slip.

Most doctors agree that mild and to a lesser extent moderate SUFE should be treated by an operation called pinning-in-situ (also called fixation-in-situ) (Figure 7). This means placing a single screw across the growth plate through a very small incision on the thigh to prevent further slip until growth plate closure. Sometimes, more than one screw is required to prevent further progression depending on the initial stability, severity and bone quality. Some doctors advocate multiple smooth pins in very young affected children (less than 8 years old) as the pins are less likely to interfere with the growth plate [5, 6].

Figure 7 Pinning in situ of mild SUFE

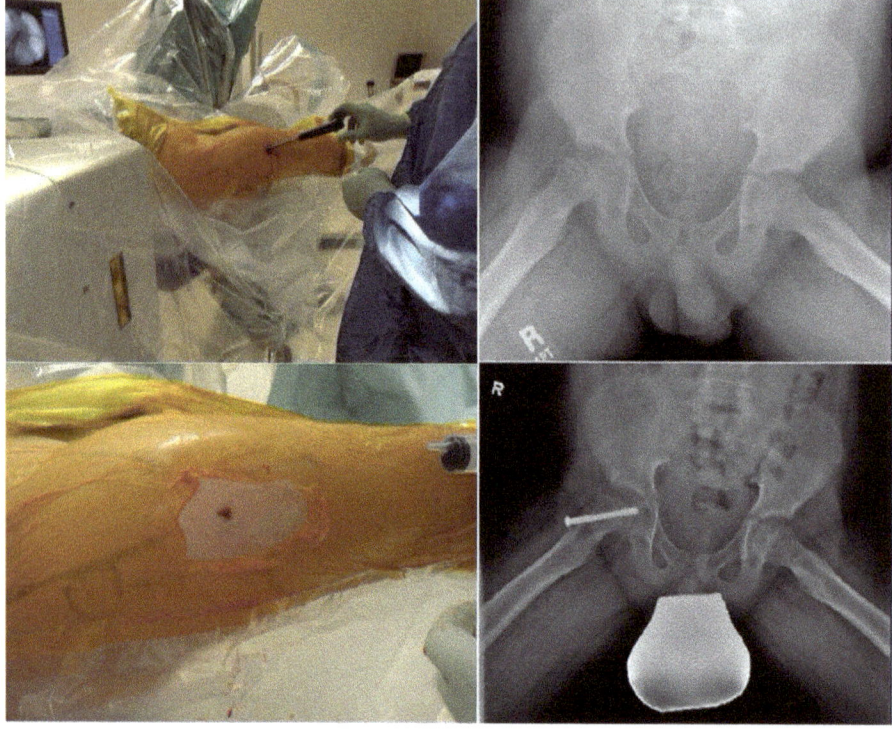

Pinning in situ means placing a screw across the growth plate through a very small incision on the thigh to prevent further slip until growth plate closure.

There is controversy on how to treat severe SUFE. Although technically difficult, pinning in situ is one option and can be successful in preventing further slip. However, even with a successful pinning in situ, the amount of deformity is usually large and it often causes problems such as impingement (the front of the neck hits the edge of the socket - see below), continuous pain, discomfort and movement limitation. There is also a potential risk of early hip arthritis.

Forceful closed reduction (re-positioning of the slip by manipulation) increases the risk of AVN and is not a currently accepted option. Severe unstable slips may improve spontaneously or by simple bed traction to become mild or moderate. Another option that your doctor may offer you is open reduction of the slip. Four operations are in use for open reduction and are named after the surgeons who first described them:

1. Fish osteotomy [7],
2. Dunn's Osteotomy [8],
3. Ganz surgical dislocation of the hip [9]. This is also called the modified Dunn's osteotomy (Figure 8).
4. Parsch technique [10]. This is used in unstable slip only.

These correct the slip deformity at the growth plate level (where the maximum deformity is). However, they differ in how the doctor gets access to the hip and correct the deformity. Their success is closely related to protecting (and maybe restoring) the blood flow to the femoral head and subsequent AVN risk.

Figure 8 Ganz surgical dislocation

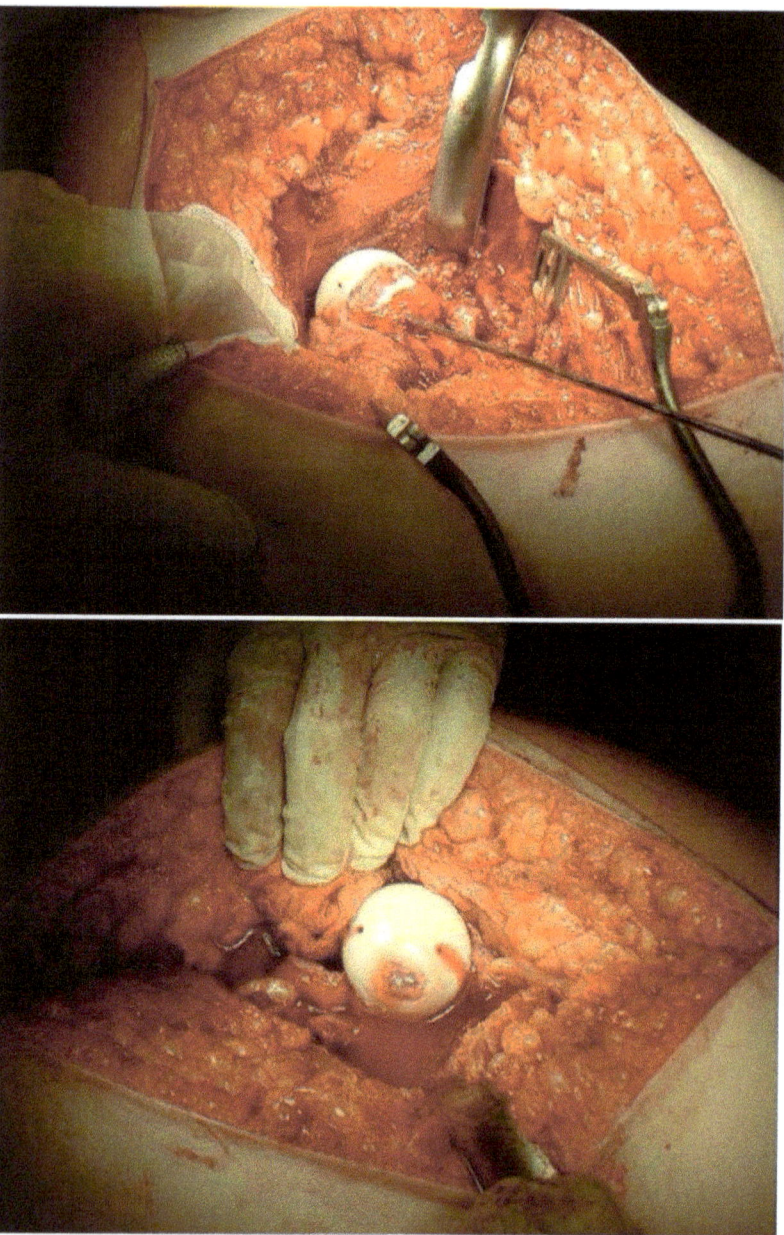

Top image shows the femoral head immediately after surgical dislocation. Metal wire was used to prevent further slip during dislocation. There are drill holes in the femoral head to check for blood supply which was restored in this patient after reducing the slip.

The National Institute for Health and Care Excellence (NICE) has issued full guidance to the NHS in England, Wales, Scotland and Northern Ireland on open reduction of slipped capital femoral epiphysis, in January 2015 [11].

The public information section can be downloaded from the following link (https://www.nice.org.uk/guidance/ipg511/resources/open-reduction-of-slipped-capital-femoral-epiphysis-476908442053).

Tables 2 & 3 summarise the outcomes of various treatment options for stable and unstable slips. They were quoted from a recently published evidence-based paediatric orthopaedic book [12]. For stable SUFE, pinning-in-situ was associated with the lowest AVN rate (1.5%) and 83% of patients reported excellent and good satisfaction. Although Ganz surgical dislocation has improved the satisfaction rate to 90%, the AVN rate was higher (2.5%) (see Table 2).

As for the unstable slip treatments, the Parsch technique was associated with the lowest AVN rate. Table 3 shows that 4 out of 84 patients (5%) developed AVN. However, you should not get too excited about this technique until we see other hospitals producing similar results.

Table 2 Summary of studies that dealt with stable slips treatments

Treatments	Number of hips treated	AVN (%)	CL (%)	Satisfaction rate [1]
Pinning-in-situ using a single screw	525	8(1.5%)	12 (2.3%)	113 (47%) excellent 86 (36%) good 19 (8%) fair 10 (4%) poor 11 (5%) failure
Pinning-in-situ using multiple pins	273	6(2.2%)	11(4%)	76 (67%) excellent 19 (17%) good 0 (0%) fair 16 (14%) poor 3 (3%) failure
Physeal osteotomies [2]	545	63(11.6%)	51 (9.4%)	131 (28%) excellent 210 (45%) good 46 (10%) fair 72 (16%) poor 3 (6%) failure
Ganz surgical dislocation	81	3(3.7%)	2 (2.5%)	52 (87%) excellent 2 (3%) good 0 (0%) fair 5 (8%) poor 1 (2%) failure

[1] Patient satisfaction results based on closely related rating systems.
[2] These include Fish and Dunn's osteotomy

Table 3 Pooled summary of studies of unstable slips treatments

Treatments	Number of Hips	AVN (%)
Epiphysiodesis	64	7 (11%)
Pinning in situ	115	38(33%)
Closed reduction and pinning	269	71(26%)
Open reduction and internal fixation (Parsch technique)	84	4 (5%)
Physeal osteotomies (Dunn's or Fish)	59	10 (17%)
Ganz surgical dislocation	70	13(18%)
Total	661	143 (22%)

In summary, mild and moderate slips (stable or unstable) can be treated with pinning-in-situ. The Parsch technique is recommended for unstable severe slip (that does not reduce spontaneously). Ganz surgical dislocation is recommended for stable severe slip provided the patient is willing to accept a higher AVN rate (2.5%) in order to attain a higher satisfaction rate.

How soon should my operation be performed?

Timing of surgery is important when treating an unstable slip as studies have shown that timing of surgery influences the development of AVN. However, the relationship between the timing of surgery and the development of AVN is not yet very clear. In a study of 91 patients, Peterson [13] showed that stabilisation within 24 hours was associated with less AVN (3/42=7%) in comparison with those stabilised after 24 hours (10/49=20%). Kalogrianitis [14] showed that AVN developed in 50% (8/16) of the unstable SUFE in their series. All but one were treated between 24 and 72 hours after symptom onset. They recommended immediate stabilization of unstable slips presenting within 24 hours. If this is not possible, then the operation should be delayed until at least a week has elapsed.

Alshryda and colleagues [4] combined results from 25 studies (a study that combines results of several other studies is often called a systematic review and meta-analysis). Their findings are summarised in Table 4 and are in agreement with Kalogrianitis's findings.

Table 4. Relationship between timing of surgery and slipped upper femoral epiphysis

Number of hips	Timing of surgery	AVN number (%)
210	Within 24 hours	28 (13.3%)
95	Between 24 and 72 hours	38 (40%)
53	After 72 hours	5 (9.4%)

In summary, timing of surgery is not critical in stable slip; however, it appears to be important in unstable slip. If possible, unstable slip should be treated within 24 hours from the onset of symptoms. If this is not possible, then delaying surgery until a week may have a favourable effect on future development of AVN.

Should I have the other unaffected side pinned as well?

This is controversial. One of the main reasons for this controversy is the uncertainty about the incidence of contralateral slip. The quoted risk of contralateral slip varies from 18 to 60%. Jerre [15] reviewed 100 Swedish patients treated for SUFE to evaluate the incidence of bilateral slipping of the epiphysis at an average follow-up time of 32 years. Fifty-nine patients (59%) were judged to have had a previous bilateral SCFE; in 42 of these 59 patients (71%), slipping of the contralateral hip was asymptomatic. In 23 patients (23%), the diagnosis of bilateral slipping was established at primary admission, in 18 (18%) later during adolescence, and in 18 (18%) not until the patients were reexamined as adults and the primary radiographs were reviewed. He concluded that the incidence of bilateral slipping of the epiphysis in patients with SCFE is approximately 60%.

In another long term study of 155 slips by Carney [16] the slip was bilateral in thirty-one patients (25%). In 14/31 patients both hips were symptomatic at presentation. The rest, apart from one, developed within one year.

Stasikelis et al [17] performed a retrospective review of 50 children who had unilateral SUFE to determine parameters that predict the later development of a contralateral slip. They found that the modified Oxford bone age was strongly correlated with the risk of development of a contralateral slip; contralateral slip developed in 85% of patients with a score of 16, in 11% of patients with a score of 21, and in no patient with a score of 22 or more. The modified Oxford bone age is based on appearance and fusion of the iliac apophysis (an apophysis is a growing centre: the iliac apophysis is located on the iliac crest on the upper pelvis), femoral capital physis (the growth plate at the head of the femur) and greater and lesser trochanters (protrusions at the top of the thigh bone to which muscles are attached). Recently, calcaneal scoring (done by measuring the heel bone in the foot) [18] was used to predict an elevated risk of contralateral SUFE. The obvious disadvantage is the need for a calcaneal X-ray.

A recent study [19] examined the posterior slope angle (PSA – see Figure 9) in 132 patients as being predictive for developing a contralateral slip. It confirmed that the posterior sloping angle is a reliable predictor of contralateral slip and can be used to guide prophylactic (i.e. preventative) pinning.

Prophylactic pinning is not devoid of risk and it should be weighed against its benefits. The proponents and opponents have some evidence to support their views [20-22]. Most studies showed that the average risk of contralateral lateral slip is around 18% [23, 24]. Most were mild slips and when treated they rarely went on to develop AVN. There are risks (about a 5% chance) associated with prophylactic pinning including AVN and peri-prosthetic fractures (fractures around the pins) [22, 24, 25].

We recommend a sensible and practical approach for contralateral pinning where the following factors play a role in the decision making:

1. Age of the child (< 10 years is associated with a higher risk of bilaterality).
2. Slips associated with renal osteodystrophy (this is a bone disease) and endocrine disorders (these have a high incidence of bilaterality)
3. Poor compliance by the child and family.
4. The nature of the current slip (a very bad slip that occurred over a very short period of time may justify pinning the other side)

Figure 9 Posterior slope angle as a predictor of contralateral slip

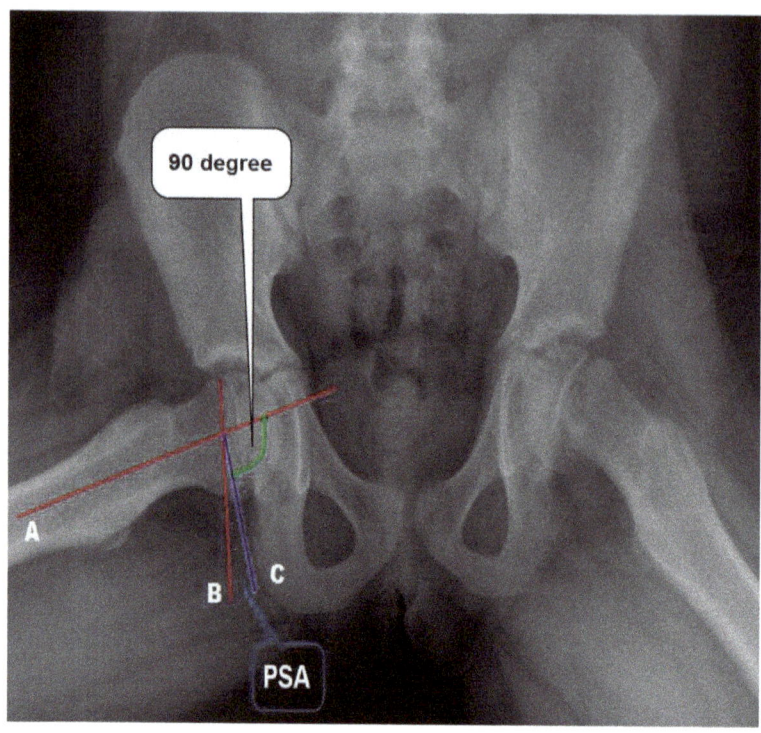

The posterior slope angle (PSA) measured by a line (A) from the center of the femoral shaft through the center of the metaphysis. A second line (B) is drawn from one edge of the physis to the other, which represents the angle of the physis. Where lines A and B intersect, a line (C) is drawn perpendicular to line A. The PSA is the angle formed by lines B and C posteriorly as illustrated.

What about the recovery period?

Recovery from surgery varies depending on the type of surgery you have, stability of the slip and whether one or both sides are involved.

After surgery, you will be asked to walk with no weight bearing or minimal weight bearing (doctors call this toe-touch weight bearing) for several weeks (commonly 6 weeks). You will be trained to use crutches by the physiotherapy team. The doctor will give you specific instructions about when full weight bearing can begin. Although, your pain gets better very soon after surgery, for a smooth recovery it is important to closely follow your doctor's instructions.

Sport activities will be restricted for at least 3 months to reduce the chance of complications and to enable healing to take place. A longer restriction may become necessary if you develop complications such AVN or CL.

You will be asked to come for follow-up visits until your growth plate closes (in other words, when the growth plate becomes invisible on your hip X-ray). This usually happens at 15-16 years in boys and 13-14 in girls. It may happen earlier in children who had SUFE.

What are the complications?

Operations to stabilise a SUFE are not free of risk or complications. There are general complications that could occur with any type of surgery such as:

1. Infection
2. Bleeding and the possibility of needing a blood transfusion.
3. Damage to important structures such as a nerve, blood vessels or tendon.
4. Risk of general anaesthetics
5. Allergic reactions to medication or equipment.

Four complications are more specific to SUFE and will be discussed in this section. These are avascular necrosis of the femoral head (AVN) as mentioned previously, chondrolysis (CL), femoro-acetabular impingement (FAI) and premature osteoarthritis (OA).

Avascular Necrosis
Avascular necrosis refers to the death of bone cells of the femoral head as a result of the interruption of its blood supply. SUFE, particularly the unstable type, interferes and reduces the blood supply to the femoral head. This can lead to a gradual and painful collapse of the femoral head. When the bone collapses, the articular cartilage covering the bone follows. Consequently, the joint surface loses its congruity and smoothness causing joint destruction. AVN can be total when the whole femoral head dies or partial when part of the femoral head is affected (Figure 10). Most AVN becomes apparent within a year or two and you should be monitored with X-rays (or maybe MRI scan) during this period of time.

Pain gradually gets better following a SUFE operation but increasing pain should alert the treating doctor to the possibility of AVN or CL. Early stages of AVN are usually painless. However, patients ultimately present with pain and restriction of motion. The pain is localized to the groin or buttock and made worse by activities.

Although the femoral head eventually heals following AVN, this may take 2-3 years and by that time the joint may have already been permanently damaged.

Figure 10 Femoral head AVN

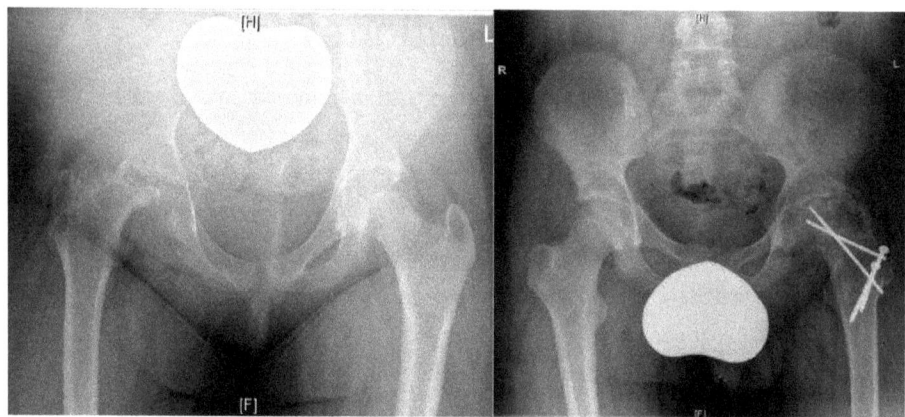

Left image shows an X-ray of a patient who developed total head AVN following unstable slip. The X-ray was taken around 6 months following stabilisation. Right image shows an X-ray of a patient with partial AVN; taken 2 years following stabilisation.

Small asymptomatic areas of AVN do not require surgical treatment and it is better to be closely monitored with serial examination. If symptoms develop, surgical treatment may be indicated. In the context of SUFE, the best treatment for femoral head AVN is to try to prevent it in the first place by appropriate timing and choice of surgical intervention (see above).

Physiotherapy, using crutches to offload weight and non-steroidal anti-inflammatory medication are often used to improve symptoms but they will not alter the final outcome.

Several medical and surgical treatments have been used to prevent or slow femoral head collapse with very limited success. Dr Sen conducted a review on effectiveness of various current treatments for AVN and this is summarised in Table 5 [26]. Some of these treatments are not relevant to AVN following SUFE and are not included.

Table 5 Femoral head AVN treatments

Treatments	Note
Bisphosphonates (such as Alendronate).	These are a group of medicines that are used to treat osteoporosis by reducing bone loss by inhibiting bone destroying cells called osteoclast. A few studies investigated the value of Alendronate in AVN [27-29]. These studies showed some benefit in reducing femoral head collapse and the need for future THR in patients with AVN but not yet collapsed. However, the doses required and duration of therapy are yet to be clearly defined. There are some concerns over long-term effects and complications. This treatment may be combined with using an external fixator as a hip distracter to slow collapse (external fixation is a method of immobilising bones to allow a fracture to heal. It is accomplished by placing pins or screws into the bone on both sides of the fracture. The pins are then secured together outside the skin with clamps and rods - see Figure 11).
Pulsed electromagnetic field stimulation	There are two rationales behind this treatment: (1) pulsed electromagnetic fields can play a role in controlling local inflammation and (2) it enhances the repair activity by stimulating new blood vessel formation. [30, 31]
Extracorporeal shockwave therapy (ECSWT)	Extracorporeal shockwave therapy has been shown to improve symptoms in a small number of patients when combined with other treatments but it has not been shown to change the progression of the disease [32].
Hyperbaric oxygen (HBO)	This means breathing 100% oxygen under a high pressure (usually 2-2.4 atmospheres pressure) for a certain time (usually 1-2 hours). A similar treatment is used to prevent AVN in divers. It is proposed that the HBO improves oxygenation, reduces bone oedema (a swelling within bone), induces new blood vessel formation and improves microcirculation. A single study by Reis [33] investigated 16 hips (in 12

	patients) with early AVN (before collapse) who were given 100 consecutive days of HBO. 13 of the 16 femoral heads subsequently appeared normal on MRI after this treatment.
Core decompression	Core decompression reduces the pressure within bone to allow a better flow of blood. It also creates a bone healing environment in the hope this will extend to the dead femoral head. A review study of 24 studies with a total of 1206 hips treated by core decompression with or without bone grafting revealed an overall clinical success rate of 63.5% (range 33 to 95%). Less than 33% of the hips required a replacement or salvage procedure during the follow-up period [34].
Bone morphogenic proteins (BMPs)	Bone morphogenetic proteins (BMPs) are a group of growth factors that have the ability to induce the formation of bone and cartilage. Studies suggested that core decompression may be more effective if combined with these factors. However, the studies that looked at these growth factors in AVN are small and not yet conclusive [35].
Bone marrow cell grafting	Some of the bone marrow cells have the ability to change to other cells including bone forming cells (called osteogenic cell) depending on the surrounding environments and availability of certain growth factors. Several histological studies showed that the number of osteogenic cells decreased significantly in the femoral head in patients with AVN. [36] (see Figure 12)
Bone Grafting	Bone grafting has been used to provide structural support to prevent the head from collapsing. Various types of bone grafts have been used with pros and cons for each type: 1. Autogenous bone graft (this means bone taken from your own body) 2. Allograft (donated from other people) 3. Osteochondral (has articular cartilage as well) 4. Muscle-pedicle bone graft. The muscle attachment usually provides blood supply.

	5. Free cortical grafts (hard bone obtained from another part of your body. Commonest source is your fibula or iliac crest which is the top of pelvis).
	6. Free vascularised bone grafts with iliac or fibular bone. This means that the bone graft will be plugged to nearby blood vessels to allow quicker and better bone integration.
Osteotomies (cutting the bone to change its shape)	The purpose of performing osteotomies is to rotate the dead or collapsing segment of the hip out of the weight bearing area, replacing it with a healthy segment of articular cartilage. These have shown very good results in selected cases of partial AVN [37-40].

Figure 11 Hip distracter to support femoral head AVN treatment

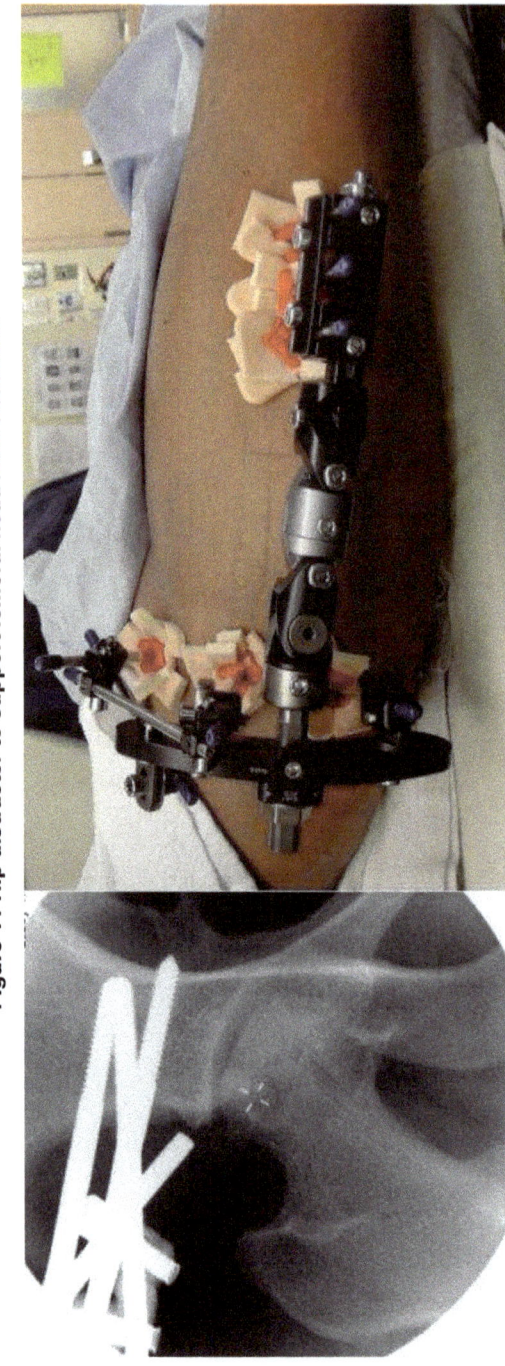

Hip distracter allows weight bearing and hip motion without pressure over the femoral head. This slows the process of collapse while other treatment modalities such as BMP or bone marrow concentrate enhance healing.

Figure 12 Bone marrow concentrate injection

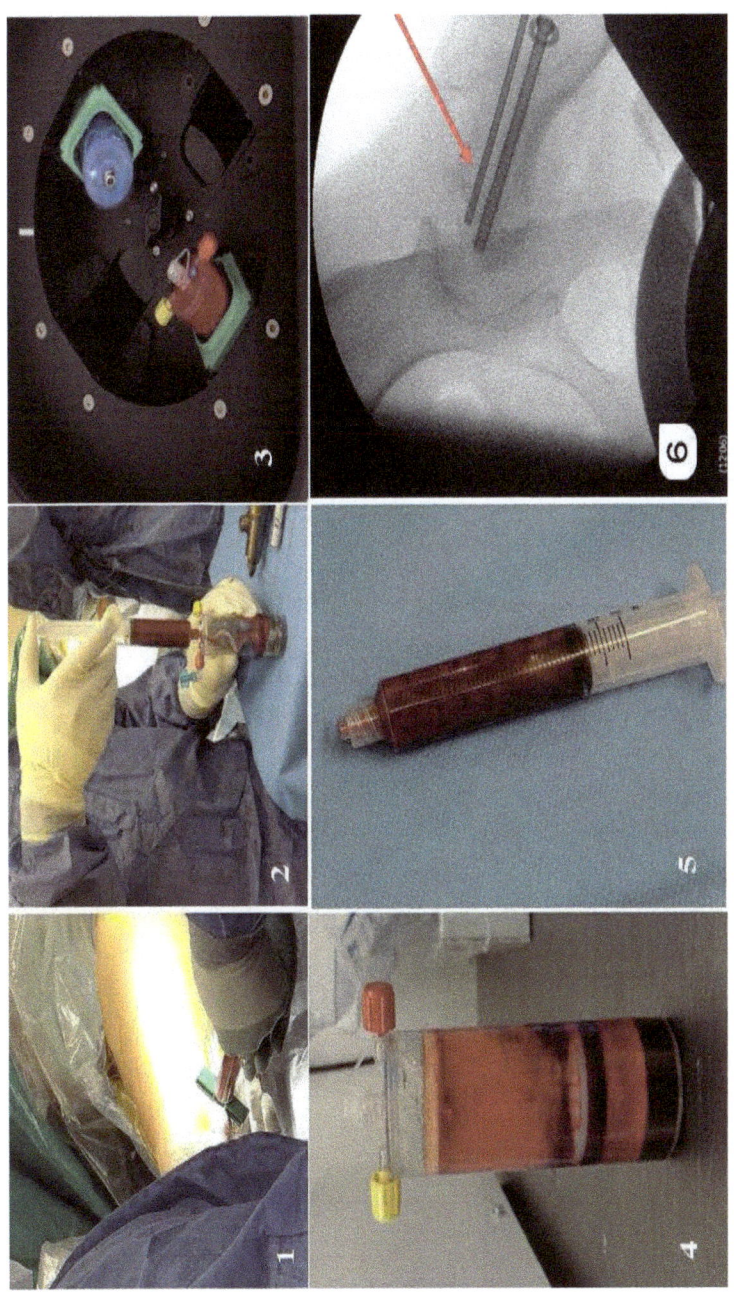

The figure shows the steps of performing bone marrow concentrate injection: 1: aspirating bone marrow from distal femur; 2: put it in the centrifuge bottle; 3: centrifuge for 15 minutes to isolate cells only; 4 & 5 aspirate the cell concentrate only; 6: inject them in the affected area

The above treatments have been used to slow AVN progression with variable success. AVN often progresses relentlessly and causes joint destruction. This requires different forms of surgical treatment. Depending on availability of resources and surgical expertise, three types of surgical interventions are usually offered at this stage:

1. Total hip replacement (THR)
2. Hip fusion
3. Pelvic support osteotomy (PSO)

In the past, hip fusion was the mainstay of treatment where the ball of the femur and socket are brought together to form a single bone (Figure 13). Although fusing the hip relieves the pain, it eliminates all motion at the hip joint. Also a hip fusion puts additional stress on neighbouring joints; problems in the opposite hip, the lumbar spine, and the knee are well known after hip fusion [41, 42].

Pelvic support osteotomy (PSO) works by improving hip stability and abductor muscles function. The femur is divided into 3 fragments by cutting the bone. The upper fragment is aligned with the side wall of the pelvis and the lower fragments parallel with the other limb (Figure 14). The theory is to increase the contact surface area between the femur and the pelvis to support the body in standing. Also, it provides a mechanical advantage for the muscles around the hip to function better by increasing their lever arms. The femur is then lengthened and re-aligned to compensate for the resultant shortening and mal-alignment through the second cut (between the lower two fragments). In contrast to hip fusion, it allows movement between the pelvis and the femur resulting in less impact on neighbouring joints [43].

Figure 13 Hip fusion

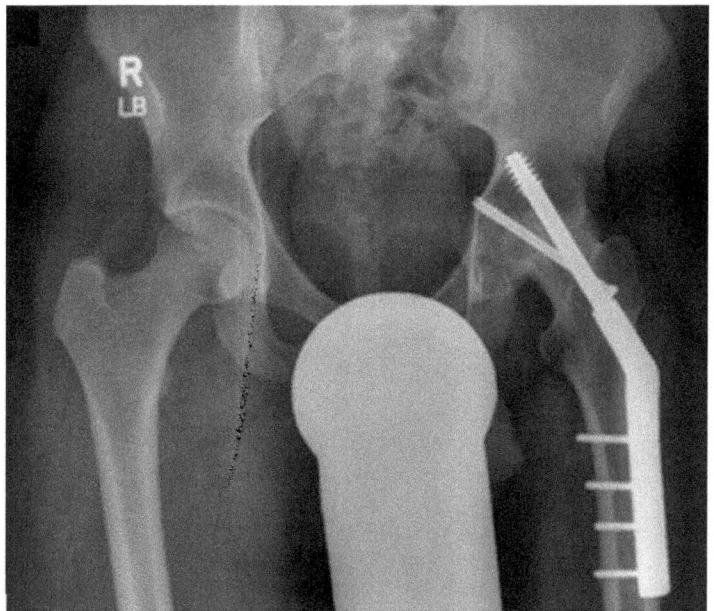

Alshryda, Jones and Banaszkiewicz, Postgraduate Paediatric Orthopaedics, 1st Edn, 2013, courtesy of Cambridge University Press

Figure 14 Pelvic support osteotomy

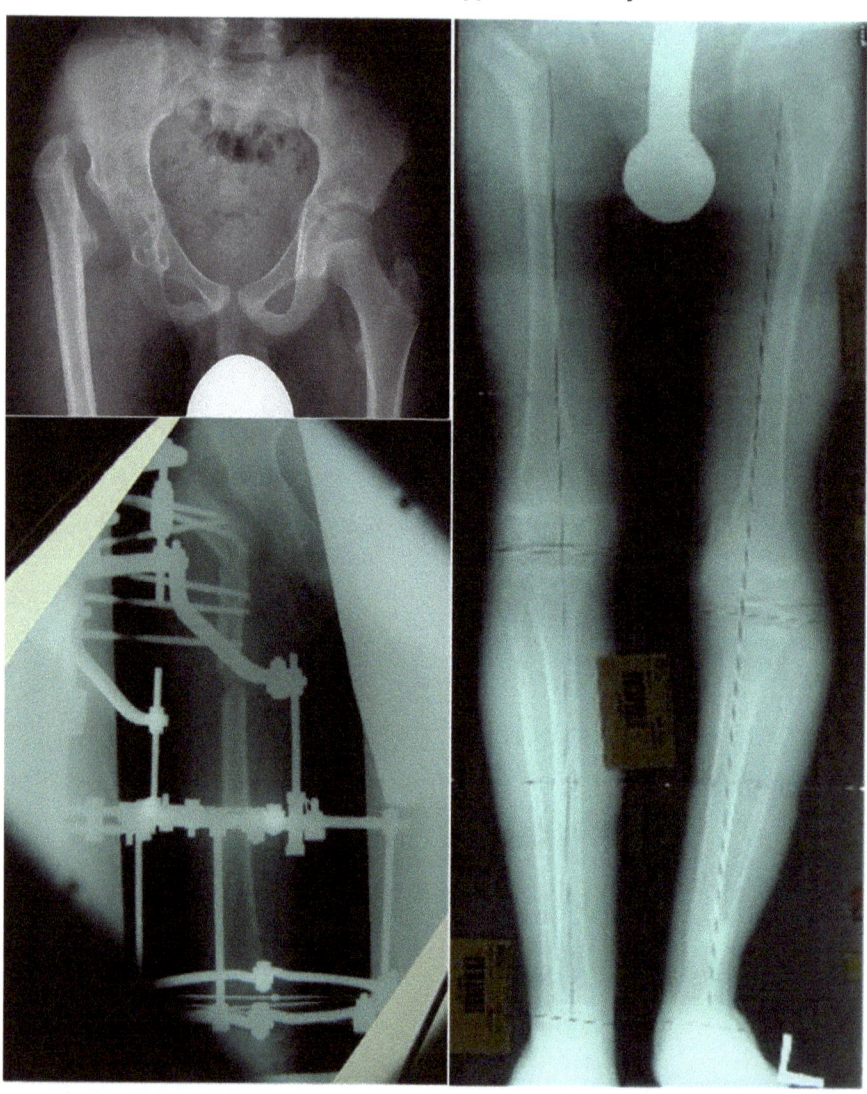

Bottom left image shows the femur was cut twice (orthopaedic surgeons call these osteotomies) to create 3 fragments. The upper two fragments are aligned to support the pelvis while the bottom fragments are used to lengthen and align the leg so it is parallel and of equal length to the other side. Images are courtesy of Mr. James Fernandes, a consultant paediatric surgeon at Sheffield Children's Hospital

The success of THR in older people has made hip fusion less desirable, even for younger patients (Figure 15). However, THR in children is challenging with several concerns about size, shape and quality of the growing bone, high activity levels of children and potentially their young age for revision surgery. They may require several revision surgeries in later life. While there is a clear short term benefit of THR in children, there is uncertainty about long term benefit. The reported revision surgery rate of THR in children varies from 11% to 42% at 10 years [44-47]. The reason for such variation is unclear. Of interest, THR has been successfully performed in patients who had a previous hip fusion or PSO when they were children[48, 49].

Figure 15 Total hip replacement in a child who developed AVN following an unstable SUFE

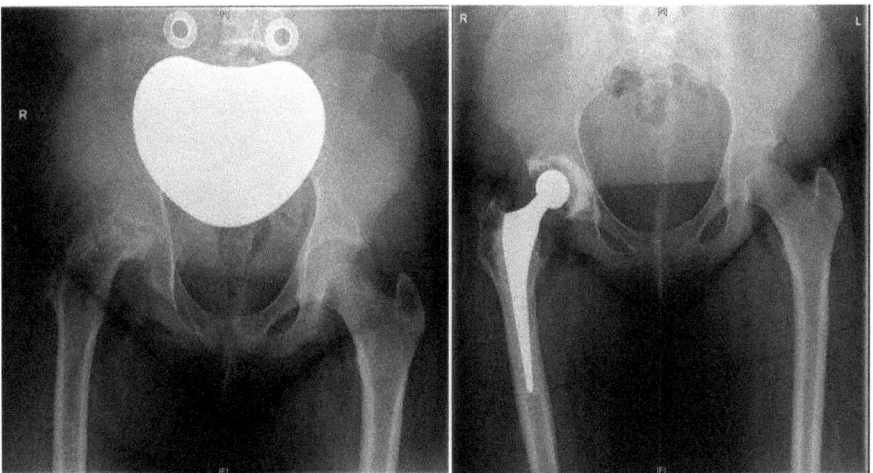

Chondrolysis

Chondrolysis means gradual destruction of the articular cartilage. This will be seen as narrowing of the joint space on plain X-ray (Figure 15). It is poorly understood why this happens. A few theories have been put forward but none has been proven. Local inflammation, mechanical factors, disuse effect and vascular causes have been all implicated. Analgesia (pain killers), physiotherapy and anti-inflammatory medications are helpful in treating the symptoms. Over time, there may be some gradual return of motion in the hip.

Figure 16 Chondrolysis of the left hip joint following SUFE

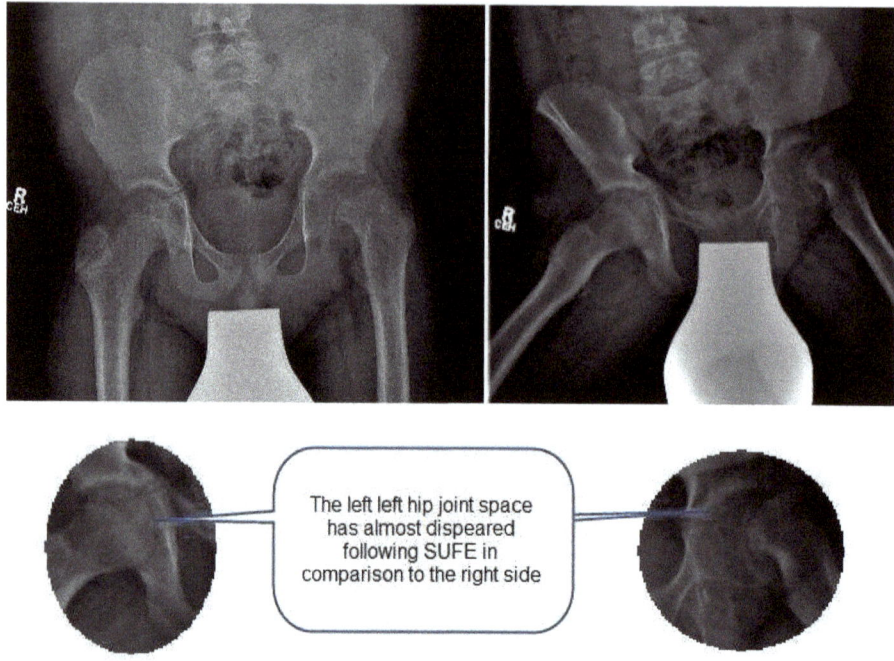

The left left hip joint space has almost dispeared following SUFE in comparison to the right side

Femoro-acetabular Impingement (FAI)

The hip joint is made up of two bones; the femoral head and the acetabulum. The femoral head articulates with the acetabulum like a ball and socket joint. Femoro-acetabular impingement (FAI) is the term given to a condition where these two bones do not fit perfectly together; the hip bones rub against each other and cause damage to the joint. This happens when the socket (acetabulum) is too deep (this is often called Pincer type FAI) or when the femoral head shape is abnormally shaped (this is often called Cam type FAI) (Figure 16). There are some patients who have a combined Pincer and Cam type FAI.

In SUFE, Cam type FAI is common as the shape of the femoral head is abnormal (see Figure 17).

Figure 17 Diagram to illustrate the types of FAI

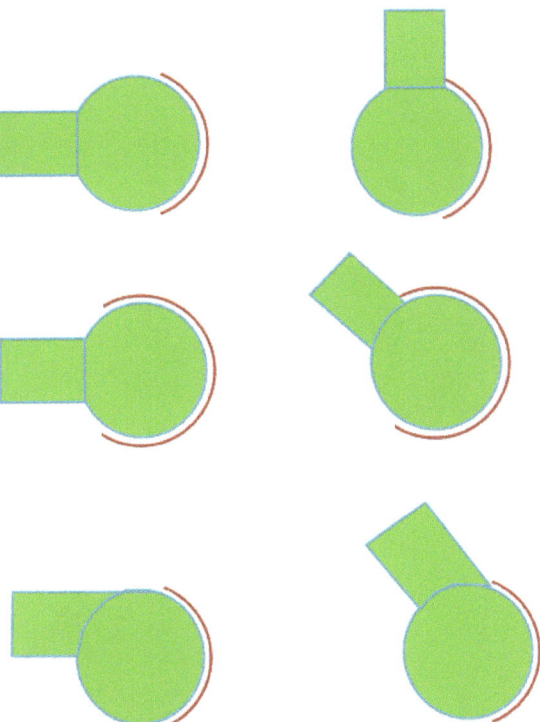

Femoro-acetabular Impingement happens when the femoral head/neck presses on the acetabular edge during motion. Top image (normal), middle (Pincer type FAI), bottom (Cam type).

Figure 18 Pelvis X-ray shows impingement of femoral neck over the acetabular socket

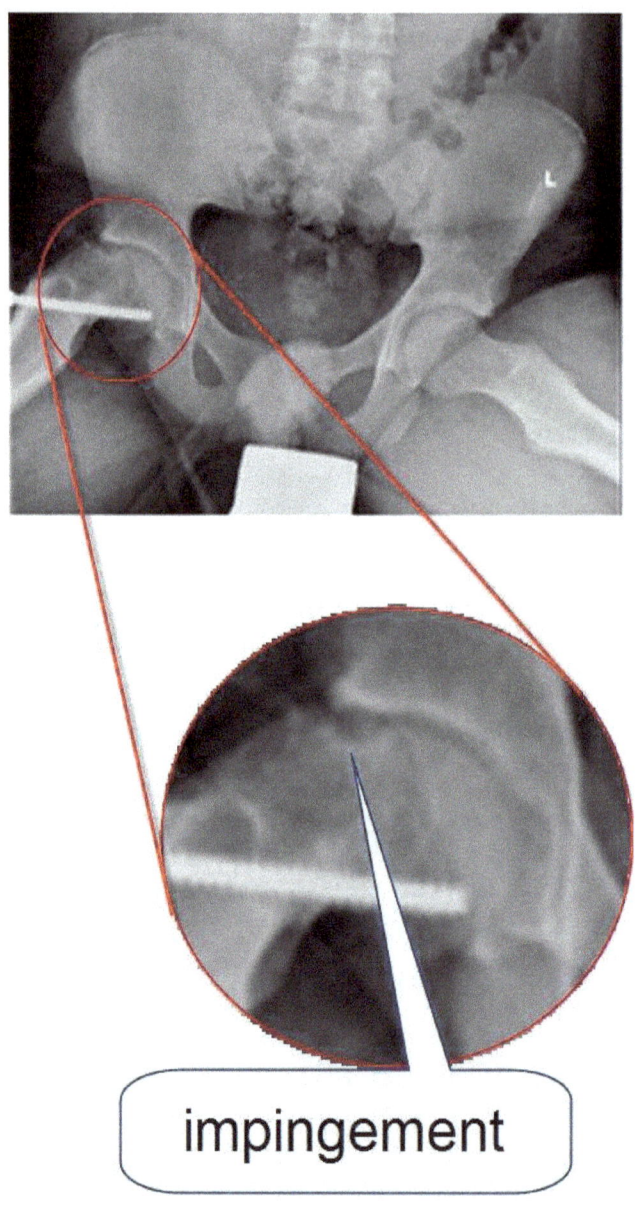

The bone, particularly in younger children, has the ability to correct its deformity (this is called re-modeling) but the remodeling in SUFE is rarely good enough to prevent the above problems. A delayed or secondary corrective surgery can still be performed if the remodeling is not good enough. Several types of surgery have been described where the thigh bone can be cut and reshaped to correct or compensate for the deformity (Figure 18).

Figure 19 Secondary corrective surgery of SUFE

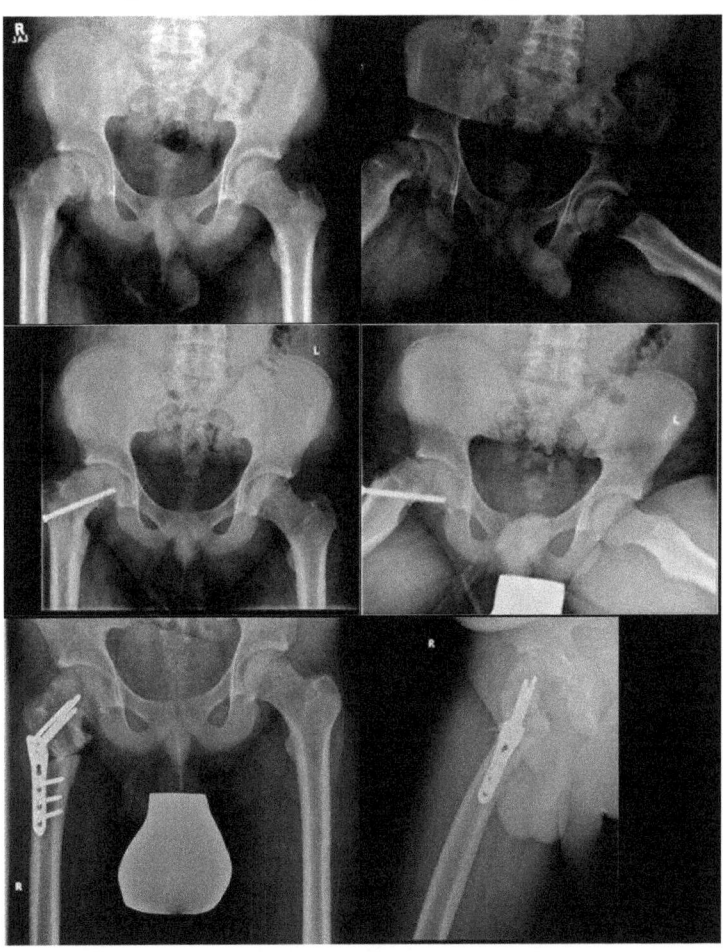

The above patient had corrective surgery to increase the bending of the hip. Before, the front of the neck hit the acetabular cartilage.

Osteoarthritis (OA)

Osteoarthritis refers to a condition when the normal joint surfaces become damaged so the joints do not move as smoothly as it should, often called wear and tear. This is usually the final outcome of the above 3 complications (AVN, CL and FAI). Once OA is established, treatment options will be limited. The three options are total hip replacement, hip fusion or pelvic support osteotomy.

Should I ask for the screws to be removed in the future?

The short answer is "no". It is not advisable to remove the screws as the risk of removing them outweighs the benefit. There was a trend to remove the screws when the SUFE was healed. The proposed benefit was to make future hip replacement (which is more common in SUFE patients than other people) easier and less complicated. However, this is contested for two reasons: the high complication rate associated with removing these screws and the fact that it is much easier to remove them during hip replacement. The exception to this advice is when the screws cause problems, such as protrusion into the hip joint damaging the articular cartilage (Figure 19) or when they become infected.

Figure 20 Screw is protruding into the hip joint (lower left). This should be removed or withdrawn ASAP

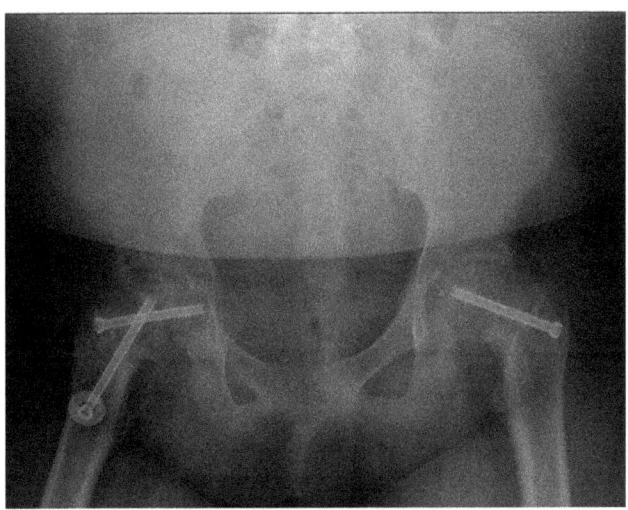

Some screws are easier to remove than others. A fully threaded, reversed cutting, stainless steel screw is the easiest to remove whereas the partially threaded titanium screws are the most difficult to remove [50]. The latter are widely used because they interfere less with MRI imaging which is a very useful test to detect complications that are associated with SUFE and its treatments such as AVN and chondrolysis.

Several studies have shown that removing screws used to treat SUFE can be challenging and not without substantive risk. In one study [51], screw removal was attempted in 27 patients (with 43 screws). The average surgical time for removal was double the average time of insertion at 51 minutes (range 26-107 min). Eleven patients needed extensive chiselling. Two children sustained femoral fractures 5 and 7 weeks after screw removal. Seven screws could not be totally removed. Several other studies came to the same conclusion and no study has been found to promote routine removal of such screws. [52, 53]

Am I entitled for disability benefits?

Children with disability are entitled for various benefits to support their living. The UK law considers a person has a disability if he or she has a physical or mental impairment and the impairment has a "substantial" and "long-term" adverse effect on them. 'Substantial' means more than minor or trivial, e.g. it takes much longer than it usually would to complete a daily task like getting dressed, experiencing some discomfort as a result of travelling, for example by car or plane, for a journey lasting more than two hours, experiencing some tiredness or minor discomfort as a result of walking unaided for a distance of about one mile. 'Long-term' means 12 months or more.

Based on this definition, most children with SUFE are not disabled. However, if you develop a complication such as AVN or CL, you may be considered disabled and entitled to support [44].

As a disabled person, you would have legal rights to protect you from discrimination in education, employment, access to goods, services and facilities, buying and renting land or property. Your parents may get help and extra support for the time and efforts they spend to help you with your daily living.

Where can I get further information?

Several hospitals provide useful information for patients with SUFE, either on-line or in printed leaflets. You are encouraged to read your local hospital information as it will provide local information regarding the available expertise and resources.
Boston Children's Hospital website provides an excellent information for various medical conditions that they treat including SUFE. This can be accessed on the following link:
http://www.childrenshospital.org/conditions-and-treatments/conditions/slipped-capital-femoral-epiphysis

Similarly, Paediatric Orthopaedic Surgeons of North America (POSNA) provide some useful information about various children's orthopaedic problems with good pictures and illustrations. This can be accessed on the following link:

http://orthokids.org/Condition/Slipped-Capital-Femoral-Epiphysis-(SCFE)

How can you help?

It is our intentions to keep this book updated and easily available to all children, parents, treating doctors and nurses around the globe. We greatly welcome help and contributions from all on the following e-mail (ppobook@gmail.com.). All contributions will be acknowledged. Things that you may be able to help include but not limited to:

1. Sharing your story with us.
2. Bring our attention to a new treatment or technology that we have not covered.
3. Bring our attention to social or governmental benefit that we are not aware of.
4. Help interpret this booklet in your own language.
5. Popularise this booklet.

Finally

You have reached the end of this booklet. Thank you so much for reading it. I hope that we have succeeded in providing the information that you wanted to make the right decision about your treatment. We wish you the best of luck.

References

1. Loder, R.T. and M.L. Greenfield, *Clinical characteristics of children with atypical and idiopathic slipped capital femoral epiphysis: description of the age-weight test and implications for further diagnostic investigation.* J Pediatr Orthop, 2001. **21**(4): p. 481-7.
2. Alshryda, S. and J. Wright, *Acute Slipped Capital Femoral Epiphysis: The Importance of Physeal Stability*, in *Classic Papers in Orthopaedics, 2014*. 2014, Springer London. p. 547-548.
3. Loder, R.T., et al., *Acute slipped capital femoral epiphysis: the importance of physeal stability.* J Bone Joint Surg Am, 1993. **75**(8): p. 1134-40.
4. Alshryda, S., et al., *Evidence based treatment for unstable slipped upper femoral epiphysis: Systematic review and exploratory patient level analysis.* Surgeon, 2016.
5. Alshryda, S., et al., *Interventions for treating slipped upper femoral epiphysis (SUFE).* Cochrane Database of Systematic Reviews 2013, Issue 2. Art. No.: CD010397. DOI: 10.1002/14651858.CD010397., 2013.
6. Staheli, L., *Fundamentals of Pediatric Orthopaedics.* 4th ed. 2008, Philadelphia: Lippincott Williams & Wilkins.
7. Acosta, D., et al., *Measurement of prompt charm meson production cross sections in pp collisions at square root s = 1.96 TeV.* Phys Rev Lett, 2003. **91**(24): p. 241804.
8. Dunn, D.M. and J.C. Angel, *Replacement of the femoral head by open operation in severe adolescent slipping of the upper femoral epiphysis.* J Bone Joint Surg Br, 1978. **60-B**(3): p. 394-403.
9. Ganz, R., et al., *Surgical dislocation of the adult hip a technique with full access to the femoral head and acetabulum without the risk of avascular necrosis.* J Bone Joint Surg Br, 2001. **83**(8): p. 1119-24.
10. Parsch, K., S. Weller, and D. Parsch, *Open reduction and smooth Kirschner wire fixation for unstable slipped capital femoral epiphysis.* J Pediatr Orthop, 2009. **29**(1): p. 1-8.
11. NICE, *NICE interventional procedure guidance [IPG511]; Open reduction of slipped capital femoral epiphysis.* https://www.nice.org.uk/guidance/IPG511. 2015.
12. Alshryda, S., K. Tsang, and G. Dekiewiet, *Paediatric Orthopaedics: An Evidence-Based Approach to Clinical Questions*, ed. S. Alshryda, J.S. Huntley, and P. Banaszkiewicz. 2016: Springer.
13. Peterson, M.D., et al., *Acute slipped capital femoral epiphysis: the value and safety of urgent manipulative reduction.* J Pediatr Orthop, 1997. **17**(5): p. 648-54.
14. Kalogrianitis, S., et al., *Does unstable slipped capital femoral epiphysis require urgent stabilization?* J Pediatr Orthop B, 2007. **16**(1): p. 6-9.
15. Jerre, R., et al., *Bilaterality in slipped capital femoral epiphysis: importance of a reliable radiographic method.* J Pediatr Orthop B, 1996. **5**(2): p. 80-4.
16. Carney, B.T., S.L. Weinstein, and J. Noble, *Long-term follow-up of slipped capital femoral epiphysis.* J Bone Joint Surg Am, 1991. **73**(5): p. 667-74.
17. Stasikelis, P.J., et al., *Slipped capital femoral epiphysis. Prediction of contralateral involvement.* J Bone Joint Surg Am, 1996. **78**(8): p. 1149-55.
18. Nicholson, A.D., et al., *Calcaneal Scoring as an Adjunct to Modified Oxford Hip Scores: Prediction of Contralateral Slipped Capital Femoral Epiphysis.* J Pediatr Orthop, 2015.
19. Phillips, P.M., et al., *Posterior sloping angle as a predictor of contralateral slip in slipped capital femoral epiphysis.* J Bone Joint Surg Am, 2013. **95**(2): p. 146-50.

20. Jerre, R., et al., *The contralateral hip in patients primarily treated for unilateral slipped upper femoral epiphysis. Long-term follow-up of 61 hips.* J Bone Joint Surg Br, 1994. **76**(4): p. 563-7.
21. Clement, N.D., et al., *Slipped capital femoral epiphysis: is it worth the risk and cost not to offer prophylactic fixation of the contralateral hip?* Bone Joint J, 2015. **97-B**(10): p. 1428-34.
22. Sankar, W.N., et al., *What are the risks of prophylactic pinning to prevent contralateral slipped capital femoral epiphysis?* Clin Orthop Relat Res, 2012. **471**(7): p. 2118-23.
23. Larson, A.N., et al., *Incidence of slipped capital femoral epiphysis: a population-based study.* J Pediatr Orthop B, 2009. **19**(1): p. 9-12.
24. Baghdadi, Y.M., et al., *The fate of hips that are not prophylactically pinned after unilateral slipped capital femoral epiphysis.* Clin Orthop Relat Res, 2013. **471**(7): p. 2124-31.
25. Kroin, E., et al., *Two cases of avascular necrosis after prophylactic pinning of the asymptomatic, contralateral femoral head for slipped capital femoral epiphysis: case report and review of the literature.* J Pediatr Orthop, 2015. **35**(4): p. 363-6.
26. Sen, R.K., *Management of avascular necrosis of femoral head at pre-collapse stage.* Indian J Orthop, 2009. **43**(1): p. 6-16.
27. Agarwala, S., et al., *Efficacy of alendronate, a bisphosphonate, in the treatment of AVN of the hip. A prospective open-label study.* Rheumatology (Oxford), 2005. **44**(3): p. 352-9.
28. Ramachandran, M., et al., *Intravenous bisphosphonate therapy for traumatic osteonecrosis of the femoral head in adolescents.* J Bone Joint Surg Am, 2007. **89**(8): p. 1727-34.
29. Lai, K.A., et al., *The use of alendronate to prevent early collapse of the femoral head in patients with nontraumatic osteonecrosis. A randomized clinical study.* J Bone Joint Surg Am, 2005. **87**(10): p. 2155-9.
30. Massari, L., et al., *Biophysical stimulation with pulsed electromagnetic fields in osteonecrosis of the femoral head.* J Bone Joint Surg Am, 2006. **88 Suppl 3**: p. 56-60.
31. Cane, V., P. Botti, and S. Soana, *Pulsed magnetic fields improve osteoblast activity during the repair of an experimental osseous defect.* J Orthop Res, 1993. **11**(5): p. 664-70.
32. Wang, C.J., et al., *Treatment for osteonecrosis of the femoral head: comparison of extracorporeal shock waves with core decompression and bone-grafting.* J Bone Joint Surg Am, 2005. **87**(11): p. 2380-7.
33. Reis, N.D., et al., *Hyperbaric oxygen therapy as a treatment for stage-I avascular necrosis of the femoral head.* J Bone Joint Surg Br, 2003. **85**(3): p. 371-5.
34. Mont, M.A., J.J. Carbone, and A.C. Fairbank, *Core decompression versus nonoperative management for osteonecrosis of the hip.* Clin Orthop Relat Res, 1996(324): p. 169-78.
35. Lieberman, J.R., A. Conduah, and M.R. Urist, *Treatment of osteonecrosis of the femoral head with core decompression and human bone morphogenetic protein.* Clin Orthop Relat Res, 2004(429): p. 139-45.
36. Gangji, V. and J.P. Hauzeur, *Treatment of osteonecrosis of the femoral head with implantation of autologous bone-marrow cells. Surgical technique.* J Bone Joint Surg Am, 2005. **87 Suppl 1**(Pt 1): p. 106-12.
37. Babhulkar, S., *Osteonecrosis : Early diagnosis, various treatment options and outcome in young adults.* Indian Journal of Orthopaedics, 2006. **40**(3): p. 138.

38. Sugioka, Y., *Transtrochanteric anterior rotational osteotomy of the femoral head in the treatment of osteonecrosis affecting the hip: a new osteotomy operation.* Clin Orthop Relat Res, 1978(130): p. 191-201.
39. Sugioka, Y., T. Hotokebuchi, and H. Tsutsui, *Transtrochanteric Anterior Rotational Osteotomy for Idiopathic and Steroid-Induced Necrosis of the Femoral Head.* Clinical Orthopaedics and Related Research, 1992. **&NA;**(277): p. 111???120.
40. Scher, M.A. and I. Jakim, *Intertrochanteric Osteotomy and Autogenous Bone-Grafting for Avascular Necrosis of the Femoral Head.* The Journal of Bone and Joint Surgery-American Volume, 1993. **75**(8): p. 1119-1133.
41. Beaule, P.E., J.M. Matta, and J.W. Mast, *Hip arthrodesis: current indications and techniques.* J Am Acad Orthop Surg, 2002. **10**(4): p. 249-58.
42. Schuh, A., G. Zeiler, and S. Werber, *[Results and experiences of conversion of hip arthrodesis].* Orthopade, 2005. **34**(3): p. 218, 220-4.
43. Emara, K.M., *Pelvic support osteotomy in the treatment of patients with excision arthroplasty.* Clin Orthop Relat Res, 2008. **466**(3): p. 708-13.
44. Tsukanaka, M., et al., *Implant survival and radiographic outcome of total hip replacement in patients less than 20 years old.* Acta Orthop, 2016. **87**(5): p. 479-84.
45. Havelin, L.I., et al., *The Nordic Arthroplasty Register Association: a unique collaboration between 3 national hip arthroplasty registries with 280,201 THRs.* Acta Orthop, 2009. **80**(4): p. 393-401.
46. Larson, A.N., et al., *Avascular necrosis most common indication for hip arthroplasty in patients with slipped capital femoral epiphysis.* J Pediatr Orthop, 2010. **30**(8): p. 767-73.
47. Lie, S.A., et al., *Failure rates for 4762 revision total hip arthroplasties in the Norwegian Arthroplasty Register.* J Bone Joint Surg Br, 2004. **86**(4): p. 504-9.
48. Panagiotopoulos, K.P., et al., *Conversion of hip arthrodesis to total hip arthroplasty.* Instr Course Lect, 2001. **50**: p. 297-305.
49. Thabet, A.M., M.A. Catagni, and F. Guerreschi, *Total hip replacement fifteen years after pelvic support osteotomy (PSO): a case report and review of the literature.* Musculoskelet Surg, 2012. **96**(2): p. 141-7.
50. Artama, M., et al., *Lower birth rate in patients with total hip replacement.* Acta Orthop. **87**(5): p. 492-6.
51. Ilchmann, T. and K. Parsch, *Complications at screw removal in slipped capital femoral epiphysis treated by cannulated titanium screws.* Arch Orthop Trauma Surg, 2006. **126**(6): p. 359-63.
52. Bellemans, J., et al., *Pin removal after in-situ pinning for slipped capital femoral epiphysis.* Acta Orthop Belg, 1994. **60**(2): p. 170-2.
53. Holm, A.G., O. Reikeras, and T. Terjesen, *Long-term results of a modified Spitzy shelf operation for residual hip dysplasia and subluxation. A fifty year follow-up study of fifty six children and young adults.* Int Orthop.

Index

Acute, 39
Avascular necrosis, 19, 41
AVN, 1, 7, 9, 10, 11, 13, 14, 15, 16, 17, 19, 20, 22, 23, 24, 25, 27, 30, 35, 36, 37, 40
Bone marrow concentrate, 26
Ganz, 11, 12, 13, 14, 15, 39
Hip distracter, 25
Open reduction, 14, 39
Parsch technique, 11, 13, 14, 15
Pinning in situ, 10, 14
Severe, 10
Surgical dislocation, 39
THR, 22, 27, 30
Total hip replacement, 27, 30, 41

www.ingramcontent.com/pod-product-compliance
Ingram Content Group UK Ltd.
Pitfield, Milton Keynes, MK11 3LW, UK
UKHW022122230426
12048UKWH00011BA/663